I0039238

LISTEN TO YOUR EARS
HEAR WHAT YOU'RE MISSING

CHERYL MOREHOUSE

© 2016 CHERYL MOREHOUSE

ALL RIGHTS RESERVED. NO PART OF THIS WORK MAY BE
REPRODUCED OR STORED IN AN INFORMATIONAL
RETRIEVAL SYSTEM, WITHOUT THE EXPRESS PERMISSION
OF THE PUBLISHER IN WRITING.

ISBN: 978-1928155959

PUBLISHED BY:
10-10-10 PUBLISHING
MARKHAM, ON
CANADA

Contents

Foreword

Welcome to *Listen To Your Ears: Hear What You're Missing*. In this insightful and informative book, veteran of the hearing health industry, Cheryl Morehouse, offers clear information that shows you why taking care of your hearing must be a priority if you want to maximize the quality of your life as you age. Cheryl is an experienced Hearing Instrument Specialist with 34 years in the industry, and she's been a business owner for 25 of those years, helping countless people in Eastern Canada take advantage of hearing technology to improve their lives. She's written this book in an effort to educate people about the new level that this technology has reached in recent years, in the hope that people like you will choose to take action when changes to your hearing become apparent. Here is a sample of what you'll learn within these pages:

- Why today's 'smart' hearing technology is nothing like what your parents or grandparents may have had, *or even what was available 5 years ago*

- What the research shows about the importance of paying attention to your hearing health, starting long before your retirement years

- Why changes in hearing no longer need to be accepted as a normal part of aging

- How using today's digital hearing technology can actually be fun and cool!

Cheryl Morehouse

I've always been very impressed with the level of knowledge, high standards of service, and commitment to staying on top of her game that Cheryl brings to her work. When you add her great sense of humour to that mix, you really can't go wrong! I know that you'll enjoy this book, and I hope it inspires you to 'listen to your ears,' starting today –this is the least we can do to repay them for their long and faithful service!

Yours in happy hearing,
Raymond Aaron

Introduction
Why I Wrote This Book

This book is the culmination of almost 34 years that I've spent as a hearing instrument specialist, and a business owner for 25 of those years. Since I began my career decades ago, the percentage of people with changes in hearing who use hearing devices has not budged, and knowing as I do the consequences that this has for their quality of life, I find it unacceptable. What too many people don't realize is that the rate of change in hearing increases the longer that those changes go untreated. What's more, less than optimal hearing has even been linked to an increased risk of such serious health problems as depression, dementia, and even Alzheimer's disease! In other words, the longer you wait to get your hearing checked and begin using hearing devices, the harder it will be to enhance your hearing when you do finally address it. Many people also don't understand that changes in hearing can progress so gradually that you may not even realize what's happening until you've experienced considerable loss of hearing. I hope that in some small way, this book can help prevent the unnecessary tragedy of untreated changes in hearing for the people who read it and their loved ones.

At its core, this book aims to convey two main points. First, any change in your hearing can have a serious, negative impact on your quality of life; it is not something that should just be lived with. Not only will you miss out on the sounds of music, birdsong, and ocean waves just to name a few, but all your personal and professional relationships will suffer from the difficulties that changes in hearing can cause with communication. Second, advances in hearing technology have been so remarkable just in the past 3 years that there is no reason *anyone* needs to suffer with less than optimal hearing. Comparing your grandfather's hearing aid to the hearing devices available today is like comparing a hybrid car with a Model T. Modern hearing technology is fashionable, discreet and easy to use. At the start of my career, I could never have predicted that I would one day be able to offer clients hearing devices to match their skin or hair color. Indeed, today's technology is virtually indistinguishable from the earbuds and wireless cell phone devices that everyone walks around with now. Remember when hands-free cell phone microphones first came out, and it looked like people everywhere were talking to themselves? Now they've become so ubiquitous we don't even notice them anymore! A pleasant side effect of this is a decrease in conspicuousness for hearing technology as well.

Most people don't get their ears checked until changes in their hearing become noticeable to others as well as to themselves. We get our eyes and teeth checked regularly, so why not do the same for our ears? One thing's for sure: the earlier that you address problems with your hearing, the better. Just as we go to the dentist in an effort to prevent tooth decay, we need to schedule regular hearing checks – ideally every two years – in order to maintain optimal hearing as we age. Screening is quick, painless, and often free, so there is nothing to be gained by waiting, and everything to lose. Indeed, you may find yourself wishing you had started long ago.

Best wishes to live well and hear better,
Cheryl

Chapter 1
Why I'm Passionate
About Helping People Hear Better

Hearing is the soul of knowledge and information of a high order.
To be cut off from hearing is to be isolated indeed.
– Helen Keller

My passion for the work I do is rooted in my personal experience of having a younger brother who was born profoundly deaf. There were three of us siblings in the family; I am the middle child, and my brother is four years younger than me. I was always very aware of how, too often, my brother was excluded from family activities due to his inability to hear. I longed to be able to help him feel included, and this longing fuelled my decision to enter the field of hearing health care. Working to help people hear better is my way of making sure that my brother did not suffer in vain, and my passion for my work is an expression of my love for him.

Let's Make the Invisible Handicap Disappear

Less than optimal hearing is often called the invisible handicap, because it only becomes apparent when one attempts to communicate with the affected individual. When a person is in a wheelchair their disability is obvious, and a seeing-eye dog and/or cane makes blindness apparent. However, because a person with hearing loss appears normal at first glance, they may be incorrectly perceived as having diminished mental capacity when they don't immediately respond to others' attempts to communicate with them. I'm thrilled to be able to say that we are now entering an era where it may be possible to 'make the invisible handicap disappear', so to speak, due to exponential advances in technology. The leaps and bounds that have been made in hearing health devices in recent years are making it easier than ever for the hearing impaired to achieve the one thing they've always wanted most: to blend in seamlessly with the hearing world.

The beauty of this latest wave of technology is that even if hearing devices are visible (which they often aren't), they are so sleek and hi-tech that they are almost, dare I say it, *cool*. There are already digital hearing aids that come with remote controls that the wearer can use to adjust the device's settings to the demands of various environments, and devices are in development that achieve the same level of customization through a smartphone app. Yes, the 'smart' revolution has blown through the world of hearing technology just as it has with everything else, and there's no looking back. Who knows, maybe in a few years your hearing devices will be integrated with the whole internet in an aural version of Google glass! I guess it's a matter of perspective whether that's a good or a bad thing.

One of the coolest aspects of my job is that I've been able to closely follow the incredible leaps that hearing technology has made over the past three decades. Sometimes I feel a bit like a veteran astronaut who remembers a time when any kind of human space travel was just a pipe dream, and now they're saying that private space travel for the super-wealthy is only a few years off! When my brother was born, everyone just accepted that he would never hear even a little, never mind in the way a normal person does. Now, cochlear implants have given thousands of children just like him the opportunity to join the hearing world at least to some degree. It's a dream that we never dared to have when we were children, and I feel certain that there are more unimaginable breakthroughs ahead in the field of hearing technology.

It's All About Customization

When it comes to treating changes in hearing effectively, it's all about customization. This is because different sound environments call for different approaches, so appropriate treatment is determined to a large degree by a person's unique lifestyle. For example, a person who spends the majority of their time in environments with little background noise might be well served by technology that is designed to amplify everything, while someone who spends a lot of time in group settings will benefit from a device that that can be precisely attuned to their needs. Even when two people have exactly the same type of hearing loss, their treatments can be customized to fit their lifestyle. Creating a perfectly customized match between clients and hearing devices is one of the most fulfilling aspects of my work, and the rapid advancements in technology that we're seeing these days make it even more exciting.

To illustrate how this works in the real world, I'd like to share a true story from my practice with you. It's the story of two sisters, both of whom are clients of mine.

It was a typical, blustery grey November afternoon here in Fredericton, when a long-term client came in to see me. I didn't think she had an appointment, so I was surprised when I saw her standing at the front desk, shaking off the rain from her overcoat.

I was a little concerned because, in the two years since she had gotten her hearing evaluated and been fitted with hearing aids, her life had been completely transformed. I wondered what urgent matter could have prompted her to arrive at the office unannounced. Every time she had come in for a scheduled adjustment in the past, she had told me how she so loved talking with her grandchildren on the phone, hearing their giggles and their soft voices saying, "We love you Nana."

But as it turned out, she wasn't making this visit on her own behalf.

You see, about three years earlier, both she and her sister had been diagnosed with the exact same type of hearing loss. The problem was that, even though they had the same hearing technology, her sister was not getting the same life-changing results that she was.

Numerous visits with this client's sister over the next few months revealed a common problem that I see all the time.

You see, everyone's hearing loss is different. Even though the two sisters had the exact same *type* of hearing loss on paper, the remedy was different for each due to the difference in their individual lifestyles. Once we realized this, we fit the second sister with a completely different technology, and now she couldn't be happier. Her quality of life was improved by orders of magnitude because we were able to offer her a customized solution that was more appropriate for her unique situation.

This is such a great example of what's possible in hearing health treatment today, and it is only one of many such stories that I could share. It breaks my heart that more people are not taking advantage of this technology, because I know the difference it could make in their lives. All I ask is that you be open to what today's amazing hearing technology can do for you and your loved ones; it's never too late to get screened.

Hear Better to Stay Sharper

Most people I know want to live to a ripe old age, and they want to do so in the best health possible. Those who wish to not only grow old, but enjoy doing so, know that they must make maintaining optimal health their first priority at every level. As people have become ever more determined to live longer and better lives, more and more research has been conducted on every aspect of how to do just that. Particular interest has been focused on techniques and treatments that keep the mind sharp, because dementia is one of the most-feared conditions associated with advanced age. Nobody wants to experience losing memory to any degree, to say nothing of the more severe mental and emotional damage caused by Alzheimer's disease. We know all too well the suffering that these conditions can wreak, not only on the patients themselves, but also on their families, who must face difficult caregiving decisions along with the loss of their loved one they once knew.

With this in mind, I'd like to share with you what I find to be a sobering piece of information. For years, scientists have known that the brain shrinks with age. However, recent research has suggested that *the brains of people with hearing loss shrink faster than those of their peers whose hearing has not diminished*; in fact, people with untreated changes in hearing lost a full cubic centimetre of brain tissue each year more than the control group. If that doesn't make you sit up and take notice, I don't know what will.

Experts agree that we are experiencing an epidemic of hearing loss. For every three Canadians 65 or older, at least one has had changes in their hearing. Unfortunately, surveys report that only 16% of primary-care physicians check their patients for hearing loss, and that means that problems with your hearing may go undetected for too long. So while many of us may need to make a special effort to have our hearing screened regularly somewhere other than our doctor's office, isn't it worth it if it means you'll stay sharper as you age? I know that, personally, I'm not taking any chances with this one, and I'd urge you to do the same by getting your hearing checked regularly. You owe it to your loved ones as well as to yourself to do everything possible to preserve your good health as you age.

Chapter 2
A Change In Your Hearing Is Not 'Harmless'

Nothing lowers the level of conversation
more than raising the voice.
—Stanley Horowitz

Because it is not directly life-threatening, hearing loss is often perceived as a 'harmless' aspect of the aging process that must simply be accepted. Unfortunately, this misconception continues to persist even among the mainstream medical establishment, where only a small percentage of primary-care physicians include regular hearing tests as part of their patients' preventative-care regimen. This is inexcusable in light of the comprehensive evidence that has been gathered in recent decades of the direct link between changes in hearing, and an increased risk for serious social and psychological distress.

In the January, 2000 edition of *Hearing Review*, a respected trade magazine for the hearing technology industry, Sergei Kochkin, PhD and Carole M. Rogin, MA presented an executive summary of a comprehensive study of the impact of hearing instrument use on quality of life for those with hearing loss and their families. The research surveyed over 2000 people with varying degrees of hearing loss, comparing the experiences of those who used hearing instruments with those who did not, as well as the experiences of their respective family members. This 13-page summary is available for download from the Hearing Review website, and I strongly encourage you to take the time to read it in its entirety, because I cannot reproduce the graphics here, which present such compelling visual evidence of the positive effects of hearing instruments on quality of life. Here is the authors' summary of their review of the research (the emphasis on the last line is mine):

"A survey of 2069 hearing-impaired individuals and 1710 of their family members reveals that hearing instrument users are likely to report improvements in their physical, emotional, mental, and social well-being. Users of hearing instruments on average are more socially active and avoid extended periods of depression, worry, paranoia and insecurity compared to non-users with hearing loss. *Additionally, family members and friends are more likely to notice these benefits than the actual users themselves.*"

There it is in plain English: when people with changes in hearing make use of available hearing technology, their family members and friends receive as much benefit as they do. Why wait until changes in your hearing become severe enough to have a negative impact on your relationships with your loved ones? The time to get your hearing checked is now, even if you haven't noticed any changes yet yourself.

The survey that the *Hearing Review* article summarizes was commissioned by the National Council on Aging (NCOA) and funded by the Hearing Industries Association (HIA), and it is the largest study ever conducted on the effects of untreated hearing loss. The title of the summary article is *Quantifying the Obvious: The Impact of Hearing Instruments on Quality of Life*, which I think pretty much says it all! Here are the authors' own words about why they wrote the article, which also illustrate why I wish to share it with you here:

The purpose of this article…is to present the executive-level findings of the final study with the expectations that hearing health care providers and manufacturers will use this information as a springboard for repositioning the hearing care industry for the new millennium.

When they wrote those words, Kochkin and Rogin could hardly have imagined just how far hearing technology would advance in the first fifteen years of the new millennium they were entering at the time. As you consider the implications of this study's findings in the pages to come, I want you to remember that *this research was conducted before the invention of digital hearing technology*. The users surveyed were all fitted with *analog* hearing instruments; similar to the hearing aids you might remember your grandparents wearing. While the authors speculate that users' reports of total quality of life (QOL) improvement naturally hits a ceiling at around 65% to 70%, I expect that this ceiling has now been raised as a result of the leaps and bounds that hearing technology has made in the past decade. Therefore, when I present the data here, keep in mind that the numbers might be much higher if the same study were conducted with today's technology.

What Is Your 'Quality of Life' Worth To You?

> *The quality of life is more important than life itself."*
> – Alexis Carrel

When I meet with clients who are resistant to using hearing technology, I find it helps to have an honest discussion of what 'quality of life' (QOL) means to them. If you think about it, you'll realize that quality of life is really a spectrum that extends from minor discomfort or inconvenience all the way to total incapacity. However, we have a situation now in which the medical establishment is concerned primarily with the acute treatment of problems that, in many cases, could have been more effectively treated at earlier stages. This is a natural, if unfortunate, result of a profit-driven medical system that stands to make more money from treating symptoms than it does from preventing disease or debility in the first place. Consequently, even the most well-meaning doctors must work within a system where acute treatment is incentivized over preventative care. This system inevitably leads to the egregious neglect of so-called 'lifestyle' factors such as diet, exercise, and hearing health care. This bias persists no matter how much evidence accumulates to suggest that these factors deserve at least as much attention as the acute illnesses that result from ignoring them.

Because too many physicians still don't recommend hearing tests, the burden of raising the public's awareness about the importance of hearing health continues to fall on the shoulders of audiologists and hearing instrument specialists, and their respective organizations. We don't have the economic wherewithal that pharmaceutical companies do to produce a steady stream of studies to justify our work to consumers, and that is why the NCOA study is so important. Sadly, little has changed since the article's authors made this statement in their conclusion:

"Hearing care professionals and the hearing care industry must be the ones who ensure that hearing loss is recognized not only for its own treatment, but also as a potential contributing factor to the successful resolution of other medical and psychological issues...Previous HIA consumer research has documented the inclination of people who have a hearing loss to view their problem as a medical issue. Consumers believe that their physicians should be the source of guidance for hearing problems, like other health issues, so the hearing industry must ensure that physicians are fully prepared to shoulder this responsibility. Physicians should be made aware of the scope and incidence of the problem and the positive health benefits of treatment with hearing instruments."

While the mainstream health care industry has largely failed to hear this call to action in the last 15 years, that has not stopped hearing health professionals from continuing to try to get the word out. This study represents a literal gold mine of data that begs those of us in the hearing health care industry to present every nugget we can to the people we exist to serve. Of its many useful aspects, one that I find especially powerful is the fact that it rates the participants using hearing technology by degree of hearing handicap. This makes it possible to see how different aspects of quality of life are impacted by the use of hearing technology for people in five separate categories (quintiles) of handicap, from mild to severe. Thus we see that while improvement in some QOL factors does correlate with the severity of hearing loss, *there are some areas where those with the mildest changes in hearing reported the greatest improvements.*

This, in a nutshell, is why I've written this book: I want you to understand that being able to hear better is not just a matter of convenience or comfort; it has a powerful influence on the quality of your life. To hear better really is to live better, and this study shows us exactly why.

Before I start walking you through some of the finer points of the study's results, I'll let Dr. Kochkin and Ms. Rogin tell you just how revolutionary this research is in their own words:

"In focus groups with physicians, the prevalent view is that hearing loss is 'only' a quality-of-life issue. The authors would agree with this statement if the definition of 'quality of life' were 'greater enjoyment of music' or some similar measure. However, the literature and this study clearly demonstrate that hearing loss is associated with physical, emotional, mental and social well-being. Depression, anxiety, emotional instability, phobias, withdrawal, isolation, lessened health status, lower self-esteem, etc, are not 'just quality of life issues.' For

*many people, uncorrected hearing loss is a serious health issue, **if not a life or death issue.***"

These words are powerful, but so is denial, so let's take a moment now to look at some of the most striking data from this study on how hearing technology improves the quality of life not only of users, but of their families as well. It is compelling information, and I hope you will give it the consideration it deserves.

Communication Fuels Your Life

> *The first duty of love is to listen.*
> – Paul Tillich

Regardless of your age, if you're like most people, you probably consider your close family relationships to be the glue that holds your life together. Our relationships provide the social contact that all humans require, and give us a context within which to create meaningful lives. If relationships are the glue that holds our lives together, then communication is the fuel that drives those relationships. If you've ever worked to improve a relationship with another person, whether an intimate family member or a co-worker, you've most likely experienced the transformative power of better communication. In particular, you may have learned how to become a better listener, and seen the miraculous results this can produce in our relationships with others. Richard Moss said that *the greatest gift you can give another is the purity of your attention*, and it's true: there is nothing more fulfilling than the experience of being fully seen, heard, and understood by someone close to us.

How do we communicate with those closest to us the majority of the time? Through spoken conversation. Sure, we may email or text message loved ones who live at a distance more often than we used to write them letters, but when it comes to those we share our daily lives with, the majority of our communication with them still takes place orally. The NCOA study was therefore wisely designed to survey the experience of family members of hearing instrument users, in addition to the users themselves. In looking at the study, we'll start with a broader perspective, then note a few key data points that show the benefits experienced by people with mild hearing loss with the use of hearing instruments. Here are a few excerpts from the end of the Hearing Review article, where the authors share their conclusions regarding the survey data:

- "...In this study, both respondents and their family members were asked to independently rate the extent to which they believe their lives were improved *specifically due to hearing instruments. Both mild and serious hearing loss groups reported significant improvements in nearly every area measured:*

  - *Relationships at home and with the family*
  - *Feelings about self*
  - *Life overall*
  - *Mental health*
  - *Social life*
  - *Emotional health, and*
  - *Physical health*

- "This study...demonstrates, possibly for the first time, that individuals with even a mild hearing loss can experience dramatic improvements in their quality of life" *(Remember, this was before the digital revolution in hearing technology!)*

- "Hearing is not only an issue for the elderly; it is a cradle-to-grave health and quality-of-life issue confronting *all age groups.*"

Now, let's see what the data says about the impact of even mild untreated hearing loss on quality of life, and the improvements available with the use of hearing technology.

Quality of Life, Quantified: How Hearing Technology Helps

This study debunks the myth that untreated hearing loss in older persons is a harmless condition.
– James Firman, PhD,
presenting the results of the NCOA study in 1999

We're now going to look at some specific data points that illustrate the impact of hearing technology use on the quality of life of the first quintile of participants – that is, the group with the least severe hearing loss. I want to focus on this group in order to show you that hearing instrument use correlates with an improved life experience even when your hearing loss is mild. Again, recall that this study preceded the advent of digital hearing technology, which has improved user experience immeasurably across all categories. I strongly encourage you to download this article and read it in its entirety, so you can see the results in graphic form.

Earlier in this book, I alluded to the strong link between social activity and overall health and well-being that has been established by numerous studies in recent years. The researchers who conducted the NCOA study specifically addressed this by surveying both hearing instrument users and non-users regarding the frequency with which they engaged in 13 activities, 6 of which were solitary in nature, and 7 of which involved other people. The latter included such activities as attending church and organized social events, attending a senior center, volunteering, and shopping with friends and family. The results were as follows:

- With the exception of quintile 4, hearing instrument users are shown to have significantly higher participation in three to four of the seven 'social' activities surveyed.

- Four of the five hearing instrument user groups indicate they participate more in social activities in general.

In addition to surveying general social activity, the researchers also asked users to rate the quality of their interpersonal relations by answering 12 questions concerning the respondent's quality of interpersonal relationships, and 12 questions concerning how frequently the respondents experienced negativity in interpersonal relationships. The data show the following:

- Interpersonal warmth in relationships clearly declines as hearing loss worsens.

- Hearing instrument users with mild-to-moderate hearing loss (quintiles 1 – 3) have greater interpersonal warmth in their relationships than their non-user counterparts. In other words: the relationships of people with mild-to-moderate hearing loss improve significantly with hearing technology use.

- Significant reductions in negativity in family relationships appear to be associated with hearing instrument usage in quintiles 1 and 2, those users with the mildest hearing loss.

One undeniable incentive for those considering hearing technology is safety. Never mind car horns and fire alarms: even people with mild changes in hearing may make serious mistakes as a result of not hearing a doctor's advice properly, for example. It is interesting to note that in this study, safety concerns were shown to be significantly higher in quintiles 1 – 3. The authors speculate as follows:

Perhaps the realization that mistakes were being made or that unaided hearing loss could result in possible injury was what motivated the current hearing instrument owner to purchase his/her aids. This explanation is consistent with the findings from MarkeTrak research, which indicates that the number one motivation to purchase hearing instruments is "the realization that their hearing loss was getting worse" and the number two reason is "family members."

Finally, the researchers also asked participants eighty questions designed to shed light on their emotional health. Here are some of their findings in this regard:

- All five hearing instrument user groups scored significantly lower in their self-ratings of emotional instability. In agreement with their family members, they were less likely to exhibit tenseness, insecurity, instability, nervousness, irritability, discontentment, being temperamental and other negative emotions or traits.

- Four of the five hearing instrument user groups reported significantly lower incidences of depression within the last 12 months compared to their non-user counterparts, *with quintile 2 reporting the greatest difference at 49%.* The average reduction in depression associated with hearing instrument usage across all five groups is 36%.

- The majority of hearing instrument user groups also showed a marked decrease in such negative emotional states as anxiety, anger, paranoia, and denial.

Given that social isolation has been shown to negatively affect morbidity and mortality, we cannot ignore these results. We now have quantitative evidence to prove the obvious: that when people cannot hear and/or understand the speech of the people around them, all their relationships suffer. People who ignore changes in their hearing may miss much of what is said at important events such as weddings, graduations, and other gatherings, which is an unnecessary loss of quality of life. The comprehensive statistics presented in this study make it clear that, far from being 'harmless,' changes in hearing represent a grave threat to well-being, and must therefore be treated with the same seriousness as depression, diabetes or heart disease.

I hope that you will consider the information in this chapter, read the *Hearing Review* article in its entirety, and conclude that you owe it to yourself and your loved ones to get your hearing checked. The improvements it can make in your long-term quality of life would be beyond measure even if the hearing health industry had the same resources at its disposal as the pharmaceutical industry. With this in mind, I hope that you will not only read this book, but pass it on to someone you know who may need to get their hearing checked. If they value their relationship with you and others they know and love, they will do the same.

Chapter 3
It's Never Too Early or Too Late
To Check Your Hearing

Don't it always seem to go,
that you don't know what you've got 'til it's gone?"
– Joni Mitchell in her iconic folk song, "Big Yellow Taxi"

Perhaps you've already noticed some slight changes in your hearing, and that's why you've picked up this book. However, if you're like most people, chances are that any such changes will be noticed by your friends and family before they are noticed by you. You see, our brains are made to adapt to changes in sensory input. We all know that when someone loses a major source of sensory input, such as sight or hearing, their other senses become sharper over time, as the parts of their brains that process information from the remaining senses become more stimulated. This is particularly noticeable when the loss is sudden and profound, but it is also true when the loss is gradual and less severe. The only difference is that, when changes in sensory input are gradual, a person's brain has time to adapt to them in such a way that the individual in question may not even notice the changes for some time.

Perhaps because of lingering stigma towards older hearing technology – we might as well call it 'ancient' given the progress that's been made! – or the mistaken assumption that hearing loss is an inevitable and 'harmless' consequence of aging, people who experience changes in their hearing seem to be especially vulnerable to denial regarding their situation. This is why many of the first questions that hearing health professionals (HHPs) ask of prospective clients are framed in the context of their relationships with others. These are questions such as: 'Do people always seem to be mumbling?' and 'Do people in your household always ask you to turn down the TV?' These are only two of many sure-fire clues that indicate you are experiencing less than optimal hearing.

Usually, it's only when we lose our ability to hear the whispers of our grandchildren, or the words of our spouse across the kitchen table that we start to worry. However, any of the following signs can indicate the onset of hearing loss, which will only get worse in time without treatment:

- When you need the TV volume up so high that it disturbs your family members
- When you have trouble hearing a caller on the phone
- When you find yourself saying "What?" over and over during normal conversation
- When you start favouring one ear over the other when trying to hear
- When you have a constant ringing or buzzing in your ear
- When you frequently misunderstand what's been said
- When everyone appears to be mumbling

These are all undeniable signs that you may have experienced a change from your normal hearing. Even if only one or two of them rings true, you have nothing to lose by getting your hearing checked, since it's a quick process and often free. As I've said before, in a perfect world, everyone would get their hearing checked yearly as part of a regular preventative care regimen with their primary-care physician. In survey after survey, respondents have indicated that this is where they believe their journey with hearing health care should begin. However, until that world arrives, this quick, painless, and vital procedure will require a separate appointment with a different group of professionals, a fact which has the unfortunate effect of making it seem like more trouble than it's worth. However, nothing could be further from the truth, and I'm going to spend the remainder of this chapter showing you why.

Get Your Hearing Checked Today For Your Peace of Mind

An ounce of prevention is worth a pound of cure.
- Proverb

If the idea that regular, preventative hearing checks are not important feels true to you, here is an alarming statistic: most hearing aid users wait until *10 years after the first signs of hearing loss* before they get help. In the interval between when they (or their loved ones) first noticed changes to their hearing and when they finally got help, they became less socially active, increasingly withdrawn from the world, and more vulnerable to depression than their unaffected peers – the research is unequivocal in this regard. If you have noticed any of the signs I mentioned earlier, and you are not getting your hearing checked, you are setting yourself up for increased morbidity in a host of forms as you age. This is not simply my attempt to proselytize or sell you something. This is established scientific fact.

I invite you to consider that loss of hearing must be included on the roster of serious, yet largely preventable, chronic diseases that are afflicting North Americans on an unprecedented scale today. This generalized epidemic is not only having disastrous consequences for the quality of life of millions of Canadian and U.S. citizens, it is also costing the economies of each country millions, if not billions of dollars. To give you an idea of the scale of the problem, I will now share the words of Dr. Howard K.

Koh, Assistant Secretary for Health at the U.S. Department of Health and Human Services (HHS), delivered in a statement on the state of chronic disease prevention to the Committee on Health, Education, Labor and Pensions in the United States Senate. Dr. Koh's words are sobering, as they reveal the true cost of our individual and collective failure to mobilize ourselves to nip our problems in the bud. Here is an excerpt from Dr. Koh's full statement, which was delivered in October 2011, and can be found in its entirety on the HHS website (all bolded emphasis is mine):

"When I began my career as a clinician, I set out to alleviate the pain and suffering of my patients to the best of my ability. However, as I provided care for more and more people facing serious medical problems, I came to realize that a significant number of the problems my patients faced were preventable. Thus, I became intensely interested in finding ways to educate my patients about prevention so that they, **and their loved ones**, *could maintain healthy lifestyles and avoid unnecessary pain, sickness, and early death...*

Chronic disease impacts not only the health of individuals and their families, but it has a broader impact on our communities and the economy. **Astoundingly, chronic disease is responsible for more than 75 percent of the more than $2.5 trillion we spend annually on health care...***The Almanac of Chronic Disease by the Partnership to Fight Chronic Disease documented that* **chronic disease causes the loss of $1 trillion in economic output annually. Furthermore, individuals serving as caregivers to loved ones suffering from chronic disease also represent an undercounted economic cost of chronic disease that runs into the tens of billions of dollars annually...***Confronting the massive impact of chronic disease on our nation's health, and our economy, is imperative to bringing down health care costs and improving the lives of our citizens."*

Now, you may be thinking that there is a big difference between chronic ailments like heart disease or diabetes, and gradual changes in hearing over time. After all, not being able to hear isn't directly life-threatening, except perhaps in the most extreme cases. While this may be true on the surface, again I ask you to consider quality of life as a *spectrum*. With social and psychological research along with economic arguments clearly illustrating the negative impact of hearing loss on quality of life, why wouldn't you take steps to prevent it? Remember, the longer hearing loss goes untreated, the faster it accelerates, and the more severe the consequences for your quality of life. It's clear that, with your hearing just as much as with your heart or your lungs, an ounce of prevention truly is worth a pound of cure.

What A Difference Best Practices Make

My hearing degenerated slowly and I didn't recognize it. I realized later that I was missing out, but didn't want the stigma of wearing hearing aids. ... I decided to try and see what they could do. They surpassed my expectations. Glad I picked my health and hearing over my vanity. I didn't realize I couldn't hear until I began to hear again!
– Greg G, in a testimonial regarding his experience with hearing technology through Innovative Hearing Solutions, Inc.

Greg's testimonial above perfectly illustrates the experience of so many of my other clients, who also didn't realize they couldn't hear until today's incredible technology helped them hear better. He is one of dozens of people whose journey to optimal hearing I've been honoured to participate in. After years of avoiding the issue, Greg finally got his hearing checked, and gave himself and his loved ones the gift of better hearing. If he and others like him have been happy they chose their health and well-being over their vanity, you will be too!

I'd like to wrap up this chapter by sharing the results of some illuminating market research conducted by the highly-respected Better Hearing Institute (BHI) in Washington, DC. Like the research summary we looked at in the previous chapter, this study was led principally by Sergei Kochkin, who is now executive director of BHI, along with a host of co-authors from the hearing health care field. The results were presented in April 2010 in the industry journal Hearing Review, in an article entitled *MarkeTrak VIII: The Impact of the Hearing Healthcare Professional On User Success*, which can still be read in its entirety in the journal's online archives. It looked at the impact of everything from the way hearing technology was fitted and adjusted, to the ambience of the practitioners' offices, on the hearing benefit and consequent quality-of-life improvement experienced by clients.

This research was ground-breaking when it was published, because it confirmed what many in the hearing health care industry had long suspected: that the best practices employed by hearing health care professionals are significantly correlated with the quality of clients' experiences with hearing technology, and therefore with the probability that they will recommend it to people they know. The study looked at the impact of 17 distinct best practices on the part of hearing health care professionals, or HHPs – that is, audiologists and hearing instrument specialists like myself. I feel it is important to highlight this research because, unfortunately, not all HHPs follow the same standards of care. However, I have always made sure that my company goes above and beyond in service of our clients' experience, believing that the extra effort it takes to stay on top of new tools and technologies is more than worth it.

Unlike the summary we looked at in the previous chapter, which is only available as a PDF, this article is available in HTML form directly on *Hearing Review*'s website. This meant I was able to actually copy and paste some of the graphics from the article to show you here, and you will find two charts from the report on the next page. This is a great thing even if you need a magnifying glass to read them in places, because it gives you a clear visual picture not only of the impact of each best practice, but of the statistical significance of the study's findings for each one! Call me a data geek, but I find this stuff compelling, and I hope you'll agree.

Bear in mind as you look at these charts that the researchers used some complex statistical analysis methods to convert their data into this form; you can read about this in detail in the full article if you wish. For our purposes here, however, all you really need to know is that the darker the shade of blue, the more statistically significant the correlation between that best practice and client experience. White boxes indicate that no correlation was found between a particular best practice and client outcome.

Consumer perceptions of protocol steps performed by HHP	Hours of usage		Subjective Benefit		Handicap reduction		MELU	
	New	Exp	New	Exp	New	Exp	New	Exp
Fit and Comfort								
Achieved Sound Quality								
Number of visits to fit hearing aid								
HHP - Attributes								
HHP - Office								
Real ear measurement verification								
Subjective benefit measurement								
Loudness discomfort measurement								
Objective benefit measurement								
Customer satisfaction measurement								
Received self-help book								
Counseling first 2 months (hours)								
Hearing tested in sound booth								
Received self-help video								
Auditory retraining software therapy								
Referred to self-help group (HLAA)								
Aural education group								
Total factors significant	8	4	14	12	8	11	14	14

TABLE 3A. The impact of the hearing care process on hours of hearing aid use, subjective benefit, handicap reduction, and multi-environmental utility, including comparisons between new and experienced users. The four shades of blue represent levels of statistical significance (darker shades = higher significance levels), as shown at bottom of Table 3B.

TABLE 3A. The impact of the hearing care process on hours of hearing aid use, subjective benefit, handicap reduction, and multi-environmental utility, including comparisons between new and experienced users. The four shades of blue represent levels of statistical significance (darker shades = higher significance levels), as shown at bottom of Table 3B.

Consumer perceptions of protocol steps performed by HHP	Recommend Hearing Aids		Recommend HHP		Would repurchase HA brand		User		
	New	Exp	New	Exp	New	Exp	New	Exp	Total
Fit and Comfort							7	7	14
Achieved Sound Quality							7	7	14
Number of visits to fit hearing aid							7	6	13
HHP - Attributes							7	6	13
HHP - office							7	6	13
Real ear measurement verification							6	6	12
Subjective benefit measurement							6	6	12
Loudness discomfort measurement							6	6	12
Objective benefit measurement							6	5	11
Customer satisfaction measurement							5	6	11
Received self-help book							5	5	10
Counseling first 2 months (hours)							3	5	8
Hearing tested in sound booth							4	3	7
Received self-help video							5	2	7
Auditory retraining software therapy							1	2	3
Referred to self-help group (HLAA)							2	1	3
Aural education group							1	1	2
Total factors significant	12	13	15	12	15	16			

Statistical significance level: p<.0001   p<.01

p<.001   p<.05

TABLE 3B. The impact of the hearing care process on three measures of success: Would the new and experienced user 1) Recommend hearing aids; 2) Recommend the hearing healthcare practitioner, and 3) Recommend the same brand of hearing aid? The four shades of blue represent levels of statistical significance, with darker shades corresponding to higher significance levels.

Innovative Hearing Solutions is committed to the consistent implementation of 16 out of the 17 best practices listed in these graphics, with the only exception being due to lack of interest on the part of clients in the case of aural rehabilitation. This commitment has built us a strong reputation and earned us many testimonials and referrals from satisfied customers, who serve as powerful advocates for better hearing in their families and communities. We consider it not only our duty, but also our privilege and our joy to put the amazing technology available today to work for as many people as possible who stand to benefit from it.

An Investment In Hearing Better Is An Investment in Love

An open ear is the only believable sign of an open heart.
—David Augsburger

We've already spent a lot of time looking at all the ways in which hearing better can improve your relationships with the ones you love. We've explored in depth the fact that the quality of any relationship is determined by the quality of communication between its participants, and that the quality of hearing is a major factor in determining the quality of communication (though obviously not the only one!). By now, it should be crystal clear to you that enhancing your hearing is all about enhancing your relationships, and that your friends and family are likely to feel the effects of changes to your hearing before you do. It should be obvious to you that taking care of your hearing health not only improves your quality of life, it improves the lives of those closest to you, sometimes dramatically.

Yet, while 1 in 3 people over 50 could improve their hearing with today's outstanding hearing technology, only 1 in 10 of those people make use of it. Don't risk losing your relationships to untreated hearing loss, as this damage can be as difficult to reverse as the hearing loss itself. It's not worth risking the love of people in your life just to preserve your pride, and that's why it's never too late (or too early!) to get your hearing checked. If an hour of your time spent getting a hearing check has the potential to vastly improve the quality of your life both now and years down the road, then isn't that time well spent? I hope you will agree that it is, and will consider scheduling that overdue hearing check today. If the immediate benefits don't motivate you, then the long-term consequences should.

Chapter 4
Why Is Hearing So Important?

When people talk, listen completely. Most people never listen.
— Ernest Hemingway

As with so many things, we usually don't appreciate just how vital our hearing is to our quality of life until we begin to lose it. In recent years, study after study has shown a high level of correlation between a strong social network and the quality of life that people experience as they age. Additionally, surveys of people on their deathbeds have revealed that not keeping in touch with friends is high on a list of the most common regrets at the end of life. During their final days, many people find themselves wishing they had made just a little more effort to deepen their connections with the people closest to them. They recognize in hindsight that, while such efforts take very little extra time and effort on a daily basis, the dividends they pay in times of need are exponential.

In light of these things, it is clearly imperative that we do everything we can to enhance our communication, and therefore our relationships. And when you think about it, what is the cornerstone of all human relationships, the one thing that most determines whether our social ties stay strong, or fray over time? The answer, of course, is communication. Yes, we email and text now more than we could have dreamed possible a decade ago, but when it comes to the people we're closest to, our communication with them still takes place in person for the most part. This is true not only in the personal sphere, but professionally as well. In fact, social research surveys have documented a clear correlation between moderate-to-severe hearing loss and decreased earnings. So if you let changes and hearing progress untreated, you may be harming your earning power in addition to the quality of your relationships.

Many people understand these things superficially, but it takes a deeper, more compelling presentation of information to move them to action. I intend to give you just that in the pages to come.

What Are Your Relationships Worth to You?

As you consider the implications of your hearing health for your relationships, remember that it is not just about you, because relationships take two. Both official surveys and anecdotal stories suggest that oftentimes, a person's loved ones and colleagues notice changes in their hearing before the person in question does. This means that changes in your hearing may begin to exert a negative impact on your relationships *even before you notice the changes yourself.*

Let me tell you something: if you still think that hearing devices can only make a significant difference for someone with severe hearing impairment, you would be very wrong. I don't only know this because of studies like those I reviewed in previous chapters, although they're certainly compelling. I know it because I hear it every day from my clients, who are often shocked to realize just how much of life they've been missing out on prior to using hearing technology. These are not people with severe hearing loss – some of them would barely even acknowledge that they had experienced changes in hearing before they came in for a screening at the insistence of family members. The following testimonial from Evelyn M, a client of mine in New Brunswick, says it all:

"I can hear conversations better. My family notices a difference if I am not wearing them [hearing technology]. You don't realize what you've been missing until you wear them. I have more confidence. They are comfortable. I would recommend hearing aids to anybody with hearing loss or hearing difficulties."

This is only one of hundreds of testimonials I could print that reflect just how big a leap in quality of life many people experience when they make use of today's hearing technology. In particular, her statement that 'my family notices a difference if I am not wearing them' is a recurring theme – people really, *really* like it when you hear what they say the first time, and they don't have to ask you to turn down the TV! When you make use of the technology available to enhance your hearing, you are showing your friends and family members that you care enough to put your relationships with them above your pride, and this will not go unappreciated.

As a grandmother to Tucker, who is almost 3 years old, I'm so grateful to have been able to hear the soft cooing sounds he made and his first bubbly giggles. These two years of 'firsts' with him are so precious, because it will never happen again – if you're a grandparent, why would you risk missing out on those special moments? I am also very proud of my daughter Jennifer and son Jeffrey, and will do all I can to maintain my hearing in the years to come so I can be sure to hear each and every witty and intelligent word they say.

But it's not only your relationships with people that will benefit from you taking care of your hearing; pet lovers will find that the quality of their interactions with four-legged family members will improve as well. I can't imagine not being able to hear my sweet labradoodle, Boston, barking playfully as we get ready for a walk. Not hearing his 'voice' would diminish my ability to appreciate his presence in my life, and while it may seem small, this is a loss I personally would not be willing to bear.

If you believe that the cost of hearing technology puts it out of reach for you, remember that we're talking about medical devices with the potential to significantly improve the quality of your life as you age. Most of us, if we want something in this price range badly enough, will put our creativity to work to find a way to pay for it. The real issue is usually motivation rather than limitation. So the question is, how much are quality relationships with your loved ones worth to you?

Your Hearing Affects Your Mental Health

As it turns out, the influence of your hearing on your ability to enjoy life isn't limited to its effects on your daily interpersonal interactions. As we touched on earlier, compelling research has shown that changes in your hearing can negatively impact your mental health. Indeed, the evidence for this is so conclusive that the Washington, D.C.-based hearing-advocacy organization Better Hearing Institute (BHI) published a press release entitled *Guard Your Happiness* that summarizes these findings, as part of its efforts to commemorate World Mental Health Day on October 10th, 2014. The full document can be downloaded on the organization's website at www.betterhearing.org, and it contains links to online versions of the primary sources that inform its conclusions. I encourage you to follow these links if you are so inclined.

The BHI website also offers a free online hearing test that can help you determine whether you might benefit from scheduling a more comprehensive screening with a hearing health professional (HHP). I encourage you to take advantage of this, because it represents a giant leap forward for hearing health care in the same way that online shopping did for retail. Yes, you can now get a free preliminary hearing check in your pajamas at home, in between checking your email and shopping for a new blender! Having spent my career struggling to bridge the publicity gap between the general public, primary-care physicians, and us HHPs, I am grateful for yet another breakthrough that technology can offer to help more people take steps to optimize their hearing.

I will now reprint the Better Hearing Institute's guide to 'guarding your happiness' by taking care of your hearing. I have removed hyperlinks for print purposes, but recall that the original document is easily available on BHI's website if you wish to review it.

* * *

Guard Your Happiness, Treat Hearing Loss, the Better Hearing Institute Urges for World Mental Health Day

Washington, D.C., October 3, 2014—The Better Hearing Institute (BHI) is raising awareness of the link between unaddressed hearing loss and depression, and is urging adults of all ages to get their hearing tested to help protect their mental health. BHI's efforts come in support of World Mental Health Day on October 10. People with hearing loss who use hearing aids often have fewer depressive symptoms, greater social engagement, and improved quality of life, studies show.

To help people determine if they need a comprehensive hearing test by a hearing healthcare professional, BHI is offering a free, quick, and confidential online hearing check at www.BetterHearing.org. Today, more than 5 percent of the world's population—360 million people—has disabling hearing loss.

Hearing loss affects people of all ages. And so do the associated emotional and mental health issues that can come with leaving hearing loss unaddressed. A 2014 study, in fact, showed that hearing loss is associated with an increased risk of depression in adults of all ages, but is most pronounced in 18 to 69 year olds.

Another study, conducted in Italy, looked at working adults— 35 to 55 years of age—with untreated mild to moderate age-related hearing loss and found that they were more prone to depression, anxiety, and interpersonal sensitivity than those with no hearing problems.

The good news is that for the vast majority of people with hearing loss, hearing aids can help. Research shows that the use of hearing aids can help reduce depressive symptoms. And eight out of ten hearing aid users say they're satisfied with the changes that have occurred in their lives due to their hearing aids.

5 Mental Health-Minded Reasons to Get Your Hearing Tested

There's a lot more to hearing loss than just sound. Getting a hearing test and using professionally fitted hearing aids—when recommended by a hearing healthcare professional—is an important way for people with hearing loss to safeguard their mental health and quality of life. Here's why:

1. **Ignoring hearing loss hurts quality of life.** Research shows that when left unaddressed, hearing loss is frequently associated with other physical, mental, and emotional health issues that diminish quality of life. Depression, withdrawal

from social situations, a lessened ability to cope, and reduced overall psychological health are just some of the conditions associated with unaddressed hearing loss.

2. **Addressing hearing loss boosts mood.** People with untreated hearing loss often feel angry, frustrated, anxious, isolated, and depressed. But research shows that when they use hearing aids, their mental health often rallies. Many regain emotional stability, become more socially engaged, feel a greater sense of safety and independence, and see a general improvement in their overall quality of life.

3. **Using hearing aids can help bolster self-confidence.** Research shows that when people with hearing loss use hearing aids, many feel more in control of their lives and less self-critical. One BHI study found that the majority of people with mild and severe hearing loss felt better about themselves and life overall as a result of using hearing aids.

4. **Good communication enriches relationships and social support.** Healthy relationships rest largely on good communication. In one BHI study, nearly 7 out of 10 participants reported improvements in their ability to communicate effectively in most situations because of their hearing aid use. More than half said using hearing aids improved their relationships at home, their social lives, and their ability to join in groups. Many even saw improvements in their romance.

5. **Today's hearing aids are better than ever and virtually invisible.** Dramatic new technological advances have revolutionized hearing aids in recent years. Many are virtually invisible, sitting discreetly and comfortably inside the ear canal. Some are even waterproof or rechargeable. Best of all, they're wireless. That means they're able to stream

sound from smartphones, home entertainment systems, and other electronics directly into your hearing aid(s) at volumes just right for you. Simply, today's hearing aids help people of all ages maintain active, healthy lifestyles.

* * *

It should be abundantly clear by now that making hearing health care a priority is essential to your ability to enjoy harmonious and fulfilling relationships with everyone in your life. Yet these are only the most important impacts; we haven't even discussed the enjoyment you'll get from your ability to appreciate music, birdsong, or ocean waves once again, and these are only a handful of aspects of the aural environment that vary with personal predilection. Another client of mine, David S, testifies to how hearing technology literally opened up an entire world that he had been unaware of before:

"On the bike path I started to hear the birds, never thought there was any…"

Like David, might you also be missing much more of life than you realize? Another recurring theme in the testimonials that I receive from clients is the expression of regret that they waited so long to take care of their hearing health. This book is my latest effort to convince more people to stop waiting and make use of today's hearing technology to get back into the game of life. It's my intention to leave no doubt in your mind that hearing is not just important, it's critical to every aspect of your quality of life. Is the message getting through? I hope so, and I hope you'll get in touch soon!

Chapter 5
A Year From Now,
You'll Wish You Had Started Today

Communication is the solvent of all problems
and is the foundation for personal development.
—Peter Shepherd

There is a phenomenon that I have observed countless times in people's experience with hearing devices, and which I would like to see change. People get their hearing tested, and the results confirm that they have experienced changes and could benefit from the available technology. They then go through the process of selecting optimal instruments for their lifestyle and hearing health needs, with the help of their HHP. Typically, within a given type of technology, there are at least three levels of sophistication with a variety of manufacturers to choose from, ranging in price from lower to higher.

Now, while some clients recognize the value of higher-level technology from the beginning, this is not the case for many people, and no amount of reasoning from their HHP will change their minds. The unfortunate result of this is that people are often unhappy with their hearing technology, and they therefore choose to neither wear their first purchase nor consider upgrading to something better. Some people even believe that HHPs are just trying to sell them the most expensive product, as if we were selling cars and receiving hefty commissions from each sale! But let me assure you that this is not the case; we don't collect commissions for hearing technology sales or otherwise profit from your choice of which technology to purchase. Rather, the price of the hearing aids we sell includes both the cost of the device itself and the vital follow-up service that we provide with your purchase.

It's like when you pay a tax-preparation firm to help you file your taxes; the fee they charge factors in the expert help and specialized technology that ensures you file right the first time, as well as any follow-up with the government that may be necessary. In fact, any clinic dispensing hearing aids is required by law to offer you a 30-day trial period, but at Innovative Hearing Solutions, we offer a *100-day trial period with a full money-back guarantee.* The goal of ethical HHPs must be to help their clients choose, fit, and maintain technology that will maximize their quality of life, and this is the passion that drives my work.

As the title of this chapter suggests, another recurring theme in the testimonials that clients send me is that they wish they had gotten hearing technology years earlier than they did. Then, within that group is a subset of people who wish they had bought higher-quality hearing technology than they did the first time around, because upgrading improved their experience so dramatically. Understand that the life span of the average hearing instrument is 4 – 5 years, and that's a long time to spend being unhappy with your choice. I've seen enough in the course of my career to know that it's not worth cutting corners when it comes to your health.

Managing Expectations Is the Key to Satisfaction

I am proud to report that my clients experience a higher degree of satisfaction with their hearing technology than the industry average. This is simply because I hold the highest standards for best practices at my company, with realistic expectations forming the cornerstone of my service delivery. The hearing technology industry is all about service, and I always treat my clients as the valued customers they are. At every step of the screening, evaluation, and fitting process, my HHPs will tell you very clearly what you can and cannot expect for results. This ensures a satisfactory experience for you, where you know exactly what you're getting for your money. I believe this is the least we can do to acknowledge you for coming in to get your hearing evaluated in the first place.

Any good healthcare provider will tell you that managing patient expectations can be one of the most difficult aspects of their work, and it's more important now than ever. The wonders of modern medicine have contributed to a prevalence of high expectations among North Americans, and this is exacerbated by the way the news media covers healthcare. People expect to be able to take a pill or have a procedure, and return to a state of perfect health immediately. Thus, the responsibility of managing expectations is one that healthcare practitioners must not take lightly if they wish to maintain client satisfaction.

The ability to maintain a positive focus while staying firmly grounded in reality is a skill that only comes with experience. There are people in every field of health care who don't have this ability, and hearing health care is no exception. I suspect that the high percentage of hearing aids 'in the drawer' in North America (that is, purchased but unused) results from poor management of expectations as much as anything. I'm proud of the standards that we've achieved at Innovative Hearing Solutions over the years, which is reflected in our loyal and growing clientele. We know that our success is due to our commitment to going above and beyond in our service to our clients, from the first hearing check through years of adjustments, maintenance, and upgrades.

Hearing Technology Helps Save the Hearing You Have Left

Most of my clients tell me that the process of getting their hearing checked and adjusting to their hearing technology wasn't as difficult as they thought it would be. With this in mind, I want to revisit a subject I touched on earlier: the longer you wait to begin using hearing technology, the faster your hearing loss will deteriorate. This is especially true of the most common type of hearing loss, which is called sensorineural. What that big word means is that the tiny 'hair cell' nerves that are responsible for translating sound waves into messages that your brain can interpret become damaged and die, cutting off your 'neural' (brain) from your 'sensory' (auditory nerves). These tiny but important nerves are like your adult teeth; once they are gone, they don't grow back.

Because of this, a preventative approach may be even more important for your hearing health than it is for other areas of health, where balance can be restored with a change in lifestyle, medication, or surgery. It is easy to prevent hearing loss, but restoring it is another matter. However, the good news is that no matter how poor your current hearing is, you can stop it from getting worse by taking steps to care for your hearing health now. Using hearing technology can help you save the hearing you have left, and this is a precious gift that I encourage you to give to yourself and your loved ones.

Along these lines, I want to take a moment here to discuss what we HHPs call 'binaural hearing' – that is, hearing with both ears. This subject often comes up with clients who have some degree of hearing loss in each ear, but it's worse in one ear than in the other. These clients frequently try to save on costs by only purchasing a hearing instrument for the more severely-affected ear. This is understandable given the cost of hearing instruments, but I always counsel my clients against it. Why? Because trying to hear with only one ear is like trying to see with only one eye; you just don't get the whole picture. Remember, hearing does not actually occur in your ears, but in your brain, which needs input from both ears to receive complete information. If your hearing test indicates that you need two hearing aids and you wear only one, you are reducing your brain's ability to interpret the aural environment, as well as your ability to pinpoint where sounds are coming from. Here are some specific reasons why wearing two hearing aids is recommended:

- **Hearing with both ears equally provides you with depth perception.** Like a good set of speakers, your brain can hear in stereo, but only if sounds can be perceived by both ears. With two hearing aids, sounds have a more natural quality that allows you to more easily understand speech.

- **Localization of sound is achieved.** Hearing with both ears gives you the ability to know sound direction, allowing you to determine where sounds come from. This is important for peace of mind, especially if you spend a lot of time in environments where the inability to do this could present a safety hazard. It also comes in handy when your spouse wants to tell you something from another room!

- **You won't miss anything on your unaided side.** When you don't hear someone who speaks to you on your unaided side, they may perceive you as rude. Wearing two aids will mean that you don't need to constantly turn your head to hear a speaker who is sitting on your 'bad' side.

- **Two ears hear better in noisy environments.** The most common complaint from people who have hearing loss is about how difficult it is to hear in noise. When you have only one hearing aid, all the sounds blend together, making for a frustrating experience when you can't sort out people's speech from music or dishes being washed! Hearing speech in noise can be difficult enough with two hearing aids. It is nearly impossible with only one.

- **Wearing two devices is vital to saving the hearing you have left.** Providing sufficient sound stimulation to both ears is crucial to prevent your hearing from getting worse. Even if your hearing loss is comparable in both ears at the beginning, the unaided ear can worsen quickly. This is due to a phenomenon called auditory deprivation, which simply describes the fact that the old adage 'use it or lose it' applies to your hearing. Without sound stimulation, the nerve cells inside your ear will eventually die, and this is irreversible.

Your ears need all the help you can give them in order to function optimally over the long term. If you have hearing loss in both ears, then you should wear an aid in each ear in an effort to give your ears the opportunity to work for you as long as possible. I have countless clients who can attest to the wisdom of this preventative approach.

The Art and Science of Aging Gracefully

We've looked at some of the science that shows a strong correlation between untreated hearing loss and decreased emotional well-being. As a science-oriented person myself, I find this information extremely compelling. However, I recognize that some people respond more to art than to science, and with that in mind I would like to share a poem with you now that I think powerfully captures the social and emotional damage that untreated hearing loss can do. It was written by a 45-year veteran of the hearing technology profession, who composed it to express his observations of the effects of untreated hearing loss on the quality of his clients' lives. I hope that you will give it the consideration it deserves.

Poem: Silence is Lonely
By Roy Bain

When at first our hearing begins to fade
Though signs are foretelling, we may choose to evade.
We tell others they don't speak clearly, they mumble a lot.
My concentration is elsewhere, that's why I ask 'what?'
Please talk a bit louder, your voice is so weak
I could hear you okay if you'd look at me when you speak.
I can hear you just fine, when you're close at hand;
If you would learn to enunciate, I could understand.
Being with family is one of life's greatest joys
But don't expect me to hear, with all of that noise.
It's easy to blame others, though it's not really fair;
It's your hearing problem, solve it, and show others you care.
He who said "silence is golden" spoke for himself only;
For the hearing impaired, "silence is lonely."

Taking steps now to save the hearing you have left is one of the most important things you can do to set yourself up to thrive as you age. Why? By now, we've all heard about the many studies linking social activity to good health in later years. When you take care of your hearing, you are taking care of every other aspect of your health as well, because our relationships are what motivate us to be at our best every day. If you want to be able to fully enjoy your family life, church services, and other important aspects of life, you will find an investment in hearing technology to be very worthwhile. I could share pages of testimonials from clients that attest to this, so if you don't want to take my word for it, take theirs!

Chapter 6
Technology for Peace of Mind in a Noisy World

There is no question that we live in a very, very noisy world. Whether you live in a city or town, in the suburbs, or in a rural area, you are dealing with a more intense sound environment than your not-too-distant ancestors could have imagined. Noise-induced hearing loss results from a combination of high sound levels and extended periods of exposure to sounds above 85 decibels. Ongoing exposure to noise levels above 70 decibels can also result in damage. You may think that you are rarely exposed to this level of noise pollution, but consider the following table, which shows the level of sound in decibels that is produced by things many of us encounter every day. Keep in mind that each of these sounds is loud enough to negatively impact your hearing on its own; when they combine with each other, our ears just don't stand a chance!

Sound Source	Sound Level in Decibels (dB)
Average personal headset or stereo	95 dB
Lawnmowers and leaf blowers	90 dB
Motorcycles	90 dB
Kitchen garbage disposals	95 dB
A jet flying low	120 dB
Most rock concerts	130 dB
Stadium when the home team scores	135 dB

This is far from an exhaustive list, and I bet that some of the items on it surprised you. Do you use ear protection every time you mow the lawn, or when you ride your motorcycle? While damage usually accumulates slowly in response to ambient noise, our world also offers plenty of opportunities to lose your hearing quickly due to occasional extra-loud events. A whole fleet of motorcycles zooming past for example, or gunfire (wear ear plugs, hunters!), or a brass band passing in a parade – the list just goes on and on. When you consider this, it's not surprising that National Institute of Health surveys have shown that one in three people in North America, over the age of 60, has experienced a change to their hearing, and an equivalent organization in the UK found that one in six people in that country, in the same age group, have experienced change as well. Please note that if you are a Canadian citizen experiencing hearing loss and you have worked in noisy environments, you may be eligible for help from your provincial workers' compensation office.

One result of living in this cacophonous sea of sound is that the average age at which changes in hearing become noticeable for most people has dropped dramatically in recent decades, *from 65 to 45 years of age*. To me, this is a shocking statistic – if we were talking about overall life expectancy, I think I would have your attention. Despite this alarming trend, however, market penetration for hearing technology has not changed since I began my career 33 years ago. This book is my latest effort to change this, because I know that there are millions of people in Canada who could benefit greatly from hearing technology, but aren't making use of it.

Today's Technology Brings Big Improvements

In February of 2013, I was invited for an interview with *Hearing Review* magazine, the full text of which can be found on their website. This was a great honour, and I'm going to take the liberty of reprinting a portion of the interview here. In it, I recount the story of one of my long-term clients, who was able to directly benefit from the revolution that hearing technology has undergone in recent years. His is only one of many stories I could share of the difference that this technology is making in the lives of those who try it. Here it is:

Morehouse looks back fondly on countless changed lives, including a man who received hearing aids from her 15 years ago. The man also had macular degeneration and did well with hearing aids for a few years. After he experienced more hearing loss, the hearing aids were not making much of a difference.

"They were better than nothing, but not much better," recalls Morehouse. "Some new technology came out, but he received advice that hearing aids would not help. He and his wife came back to me, but my experience told me that the new technology was worth a try."

Morehouse was right, and she and her long-time customer were able to sit across a table from each other and have a normal conversation. "I was so grateful he tried the new technology," says Morehouse. "His wife was losing her voice because of having to raise it for him. After he got the new technology, he was able to go walking alone, which he had not done in years."

It is so inspiring to see people's lives change for the better in this way, and today's technology is allowing my work to have an even greater impact. It really is true that, like this gentleman, even people whose hearing technology is only a few years old can experience major improvements by taking advantage of the innovations that have happened in just the past five years. In the next section, I'll share some of the cutting-edge trends that I find to be the most exciting. Sometimes even I can't believe what's possible now, because it's all happened so fast!

"There's An App For That"

If you know what this section's title refers to, then you've probably already jumped on the latest technology bandwagon. But if you don't, let me fill you in: the word 'app' refers to the innumerable little software programs that are created for today's 'smart' phones and tablets. These apps have been developed for every purpose you can think of, from entertainment to financial planning to ordering takeout, and a zillion other purposes that might never occur to you. Among these is an app that actually gives you the ability to customize the settings of your hearing technology with the tap of a finger. If you don't believe me, then take it from the geeks at www.techradar.com, a UK-based technology trend-watching e-magazine. They note in their article (entitled *iPods to Ear Pods: Smartphones Are Supercharging Hearing Aids*) that this technology is currently only available for iPhones, but that similar technology for other smartphone platforms is under development. I've bolded the text in a few places for emphasis.

* * *

The amount of hearing aids being used in people of working age, combined with an increase of the average age of the smartphone user, means the time has finally come to integrate the two technologies.

Prior to products like the LiNX and Halo combining with newer iPhones, iPod touch models or iPads, users would need to carry or install cumbersome extra accessories like a wireless pendant or phone clip to allow phones to speak to the hearing aids.

*The strength of combining a hearing aid with a smartphone is the **fact it removes so many other tools previously needed to improve hearing technology.** Not only can you stream music directly from* *your iDevice [iPhone, iPod, or iPad], but users can get tailored programs to improve their ability to hear in different environments.*

For instance, listening to someone in a quiet room and noisy restaurant needs different levels of noise suppression, which would have previously required fiddling with the units behind the ear or using a dedicated remote control. **Now it's a simple as a tap on the screen, meaning users don't even have to admit to having a hearing impairment – instead, it can be put down to today's acceptance of antisocial phone fiddling.**

The smartphone also brings other benefits – it's packed with sensors that can benefit hearing aid users. **Using GPS, they can geotag an area with a certain set of settings and be prompted to activate them when re-entering the same place.**

The smartphone's display also helps save a great deal of money too, according to Shiraz.

"The best feature response I've seen for the Halo is 'Find my hearing aid'. The price of these hearing aids is not cheap by any means, and one of nicest things people found is, **if they've lost their hearing aids and it would normally cost a few thousand to get more, the finder feature shows where they were last seen, giving the postcode indication.**

"But if they're nearby and turned on, the Bluetooth LE connection shows bars that get 'hot and cold' depending on how close you are."

* * *

Now, it's true that the price point for iPhone-compatible hearing technology is at the upper end of the spectrum. However, you may decide that the benefits are worth it if you're an iPhone user. I can tell you that a surprising number of people do manage to lose their expensive hearing technology at some point, and those folks will tell you that the 'find my hearing aid' feature is worth the investment on its own.

The Wireless Revolution: Not Just For Geeks Anymore!

There's no question that the 'smart' revolution in hearing technology is exciting stuff. However, if you're not a smartphone fan or the price puts you off, there is a great selection of hearing technology on the market that can offer almost everything that the smartphone devices can – they just require a little extra equipment to do it. Most commonly, this consists of a small device worn around the neck (the article above refers to these as pendants, but they're really remote controls), which allows you to adjust the settings of your in-ear technology. These remotes mediate between your earpiece and any wireless-enabled devices that you wish to connect with, using the same technology that allows people to wirelessly talk on their cell phones, navigate their computers, and play music from an MP3 device in their cars.

Almost all cell phones come equipped with this wireless capability these days, even the non-'smart' models. It allows a caller's voice to be delivered directly into your ear, and gives you two volume controls: one on your phone, and one on your remote. There are also landline phones available now that are wireless-enabled, allowing you to make landline calls using your hearing technology as well. Since the wireless revolution has swept through every aspect of the consumer electronics market, newer televisions can also be integrated with your hearing instruments, meaning that the sound from the set is sent directly to your earpiece via wireless transmission. Now, not only will your family members not have to ask you to turn down the TV, they may need to ask you to turn it *up* if they want to watch as well! The same applies to your computers and tablets; you can stream audio from them directly into your earpiece, allowing you to watch movies or teleconference with ease.

These wireless features are neat enough on their own, but they still represent only a fraction of what's possible with today's technology. In the next section, we'll get down to the main purpose of all hearing technology: helping you hear better in noisy environments.

Creating Order from Chaos: Noise Reduction in Hearing Technology

If you're inclined to pursue further reading on the exciting breakthroughs that are happening every day now in hearing technology, my fellow Canadian Peter Stelmacovich keeps an informative and entertaining blog entitled *Deafened But Not Silent: How to Live Life to the Max with Hearing Loss*. As you might guess, Peter likes to have fun – he's a dedicated amateur rock musician, among other things. Perhaps most remarkably, however, he is a practicing audiologist who also happens to be functionally deaf. I often click over to his blog when I have a free moment and am looking for some insight and inspiration.

In February 2013, Peter wrote a post entitled *Best Ways to Hear Better in Noise*, which offers a comprehensive yet streamlined look at how different types of hearing technology cope with noisy environments. In it, he goes into more detail than I have space for here, but I'd like to reprint the first part of that post at least, to give you an idea of what today's hearing technology is designed to do for you. As you read it, ask yourself whether hearing a person speak is challenging for you in noisy situations. If the answer is yes, then you'll be surprised at how much today's technology can help.

* * *

Hearing loss results in two main problems; loss of audibility, and loss of clarity in noise.

Loss of Audibility. *This means that sounds are too soft to hear. We have a couple of strategies to make sounds more audible.*

1. *Amplification. Today's modern hearing aids selectively make softer sounds louder than louder sounds.*

2. *Frequency Compression. In some hearing aids such as the ones provided by my company, Phonak, the hearing aid can shift high-pitched sounds down to lower pitches. The logic is that you may have too much damage in the high pitches to amplify the sounds sufficiently, so we will shift these sounds to regions where you have better hearing.*

3. *Cochlear Implants. If high-powered hearing aids equipped with frequency compression no longer help you hear, we now turn to a Cochlear Implant to make sound audible.*

Loss of Clarity in Noise. *I wish that hearing loss were merely a problem of loss of audibility. It would be so much easier just to amplify the sounds and be done with it. Just like wearing a pair of corrective lenses for vision, right? Wrong.*

After we do our best to make sound audible, we also have to do something about getting rid of the background noise. As one's hearing loss gets worse, not only do we need stronger and stronger hearing aids, but we also need to get rid of more and more noise. For example, a person with normal hearing can handle a signal-to-noise (SNR) ratio of 0 and still understand most of what is being said. An SNR of 0 means that the person talking to you is the same loudness as the person you don't want to listen to. This happens all the time. Imagine a restaurant. There are people all around you talking at the same loudness as your significant other across from you. You normal hearing folks can handle this, people with hearing loss cannot.

I should mention here that not all hearing instruments are created equal, so when you are comparing hearing devices, you need to be sure that the models you are comparing all share the same features and capabilities. You want to narrow down the features you need with your HHP first, and then begin to compare the models offered by different manufacturers within that category. Remember that your hearing loss is unique to you just like your fingerprints, so if a particular instrument works or doesn't work for someone else, that doesn't mean you'll have the same experience with it.

This is only the beginning of a conversation that you need to have first with yourself, and then with a qualified hearing health professional: is my ability to hear compromised in noisy environments? Is this causing me to miss out on important aspects of my life? If the answer is yes (or even maybe), then I hope you'll take advantage of the incredible technology that's available to help you start hearing better, today.

Conclusion
Don't Just Read This, Take Action!

First, I want to thank you for taking the time to read my little book all the way through. Just by doing that, you've shown that you're committed to addressing changes in your hearing as soon as they appear, and this is an admirable thing. I very much hope that this book has inspired you to get your hearing tested early and often – at least as often as you get a routine physical exam. This is the crucial first step to reap the benefits of optimal hearing now and in the future, when it may matter most.

Your quality of life doesn't have to suffer when your hearing starts to go. There are so many options available for treatment, but you need to be proactive if you want to preserve the hearing you have left for as long as possible. I've said it before, and I'll say it again: when it's left untreated, hearing loss only gets worse, not better. The first step is to get a hearing test every two years. The second is to acknowledge that you need help if you suspect that your hearing has changed, and take steps to get the quality professional support you need. At Innovative Hearing Solutions, we provide the following as an integral part of our audiology and hearing instrument-fitting practice:

- Professionalism and Top-Level Service – Your Happiness is Our Goal
- Experienced and Knowledgeable Staff
- Warm and Friendly Atmosphere
- Convenient Locations in New Brunswick and Nova Scotia
- Hearing-Enhancement Discovery Process

- Private, Customized Treatment Plans
- A Comprehensive Toolkit to Ensure Your Success
- Fully refundable 100-day trial period for all devices
- Tinnitus consulting
- We Work With All Third-Party Payers

If you suspect that you or someone you love may have experienced changes in hearing, don't hesitate to contact us today. We will do all we can to make the discovery process, testing, diagnosis, hearing aid fitting, and follow-up care as seamless as possible. We want to be there for you, our clients, to inspire you to get hearing devices that suit your lifestyle and budget, and it's our great joy to watch the transformation that can happen when clients are committed to their hearing health. Change is so hard for most of us, and we want to make sure you are successful in your hearing journey, and that you get the most out of life by keeping active with more confidence by hearing the best you can in all situations.

Innovative Hearing Solutions has a referral card that we hand out to our many satisfied customers. It says that we believe that conversation is one of life's greatest pleasures, and that everyone deserves to be able to enjoy it. Hearing loss should not be looked at as a disability, but as something that requires engaging in the world in a special way. We must find a way to approach the problem differently, the card says. We must make hearing health care be about reconnecting with family and friends and making every moment count, not about 'living with a disability.' This card carries our core message into the communities that our clinics serve, inspiring people to take care of their relationships and quality of life by taking care of their hearing. The vast majority of our clients are delighted to help us spread the word, because they have personally experienced the difference that hearing technology has made in their lives.

I'd like to take this opportunity to acknowledge the honour and privilege that Innovative Hearing Solutions has had to serve hundreds of our nation's veterans over the years. They served our country - it is our turn to serve them. We have also processed hundreds of worker's compensation claims, helping people access the resources in support of their hearing health.

Rather than providing over-the-counter sales or a one-solution-fits-all approach, at Innovative Hearing Solutions we do everything in our power to maximize our clients' results through top-level care and customization, from the very first consultation. We love to get to know our clients, and I especially enjoy making people laugh! You deserve to enjoy the quality of life that improved hearing brings, and you deserve a hearing health care experience that surpasses your expectations. Hearing technology can help you reclaim the pieces of your life that you thought were gone for good, and your loved ones will be grateful to have you back as well. It really is a win-win, and I hope this book has inspired you to take care of your hearing health, today and tomorrow.

We want to hear your stories about your hearing journeys.
Please mail them to one of our locations or email them to
hearing@nbnet.nb.ca.
Website www.hearingservices.ca

www.ingramcontent.com/pod-product-compliance
Lightning Source LLC
Chambersburg PA
CBHW070258290326
41930CB00041B/2637